Eat Right For Your Blood Type

A Guide to Healthy Blood Type Diet

*Understand What to Eat
According to Your Blood Type*

By

I0837548

WaraWaran R.

Pawana Publishing Inc.

A wise man once said...
To eat is a necessity, but to eat intelligently is an art
- Francois de la Rochefoucauld

First Publish in 2015 by Pawana Publishing Inc.

Copyright © 2015 by Warawaran Roongruangsri

All rights reserved.

No part of this publication may be reproduced or distribute in any form or by means, electronic or mechanical, or stored in database or retrieval system without prior written from the publisher.

ISBN 978-1514276945

This document is geared towards providing exact and reliable information in regards to the topic and issue covered. The publication is sold with the idea that the publisher is not required to render accounting, officially permitted, or otherwise, qualified services. If advice is necessary, legal or professional, a practiced individual in the profession should be ordered.

- From a Declaration of Principles which was accepted and approved equally by a Committee of the American Bar Association and a Committee of Publishers and Associations.

In no way is it legal to reproduce, duplicate, or transmit any part of this document in either electronic means or in printed format. Recording of this publication is strictly prohibited and any storage of this document is not allowed unless with written permission from the publisher. All rights reserved.

The information provided herein is stated to be truthful and consistent, in that any liability, in terms of inattention or otherwise, by any usage or abuse of any policies, processes, or directions contained within is the solitary and utter responsibility of the recipient reader. Under no circumstances will any legal responsibility or blame be held against the publisher for any reparation, damages, or monetary loss due to the information herein, either directly or indirectly.

Respective authors own all copyrights not held by the publisher.

The information herein is offered for informational purposes solely, and is universal as so. The presentation of the information is without contract or any type of guarantee assurance.

The trademarks that are used are without any consent, and the publication of the trademark is without permission or backing by the trademark owner. All trademarks and brands within this book are for clarifying purposes only and are the owned by the owners themselves, not affiliated with this document.

Table of Contents

AUTHOR'S NOTE

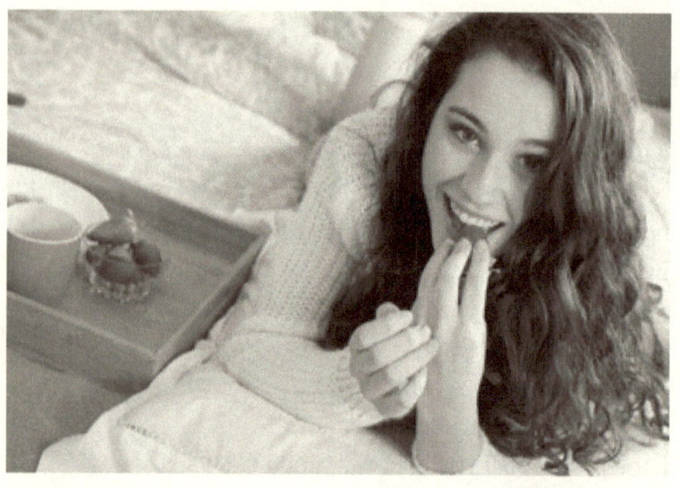

I want to thank you and congratulate you for downloading the book, "Eat Right For Your Blood Type: *A Guide to Healthy Blood Type Diet, Understand What to Eat According to Your Blood Type*".

This book contains information on the Eating Right For Your Blood Type Guide and the Blood Type Diet which also proven steps and strategies on how to make it work so you can get the results that you want.

Among all the diets and other weight loss trends and fads out there, the Blood Type Diet stands out. Find out what it is all about and how it works in effectively helping you lose weight and become younger, stronger and healthier!

Thanks again for downloading this book, A little knowledge can change your life.

I hope you enjoy it!.

WaraWara R.

Chapter 1 - An Introduction to the Blood Type Diet

In the past, the word "diet" was mainly seen as a method to lose weight or shed off a few inches and pounds. However, as time passed, more and more people are growing to appreciate the other health benefits of observing a proper diet. This explains the increasing number of various types of diets that are being introduced today, with each diet claiming to provide better results, and with less effort, to boot.

Among this sea of health and weight loss diets is the Blood Type Diet, which basically operates on the premise that the different blood types of humans have corresponding foods and exercises suitable to them. In short, the blood type of a person determines how his or her body responds to certain food.

The Blood Type and Food Connection

As proven by other diets over and over again, not everyone responds to the same diet in the same way. There are those that may find a specific diet working for them, but there are those who may find it ineffective. This is largely because of the variability of the body's chemistry, and it also explains the connection between one's blood type and diet, when taken in the context of the Blood Type Diet.

In a room filled with people, majority possess a blood type of O. There are those who belong to the blood type A and B, respectively. Meanwhile, one or two may have blood type AB, which is quite rare. Not all these people will respond to the same type of food, and their blood types also have something to do with that.

The four blood types - A, B, AB and O - are distinguished by the antigens, or immune defense systems that are on the surface of the red blood cells. Over time, these blood types have become known to act as a defense against certain diseases or illnesses. For example, several researches have revealed that those that belong to the O blood type have lower risks of heart attacks.

The blood type of a person tells a lot about his body chemistry. It is considered to be a vital tool for understanding how your body reacts to various types of food, its susceptibility to different types of illnesses, as well as your natural reaction to stress and other similar triggers. In fact, you can liken it to your fingerprint, as it gives you a unique identity and represents a biochemical makeup that is distinctly yours.

For instance, when it comes to food, Type O individuals will absorb the nutrients from certain foods differently compared to when Type A or Type B individuals ingest the exact same type of foods, and vice versa.

Similarly, a person with blood type O is likely to respond faster to a specific set of exercises than when one with blood type AB will also undertake the regimen.

Of course, the Blood Type Diet is not without its critics and detractors. According to some medical experts, the blood type and food choices really have nothing to do with each other, as long as you maintain a healthy digestive system and adhere to clean and healthy living habits.

Application of the Blood Type Diet

According to naturopathy experts and advocates of the Blood Type Diet, people's susceptibility to certain illnesses and medical conditions are directly related to the blood group they belong in. Thus, the type and amount of exercise that one should get should also be in accordance to what that blood type requires. The same principle applies to the foods they should eat and the general diet they ought to follow.

This diet can be followed by people of all ages, instead of being limited to specific age groups or even blood groups.

When following the Blood Type Diet, one must be cognizant of the fact that not all persons are the same. The mere fact that they have different blood types is already more than enough indication that they will also have to adhere to different diets and exercise programs. What worked for your friend may not work for you, since you do not necessarily belong to the same blood group.

- Know what your blood type is. Before you can get started on this diet, you must first make sure what blood group you belong to. As mentioned earlier, there are four blood groups: A, B, AB and O.

- In a nutshell, find out which foods are most suitable for your blood group. We will be going into more detail on the appropriate diets for each blood group later in this book, but for now, here is a quick rundown of the main types of food they should eat.

> Blood Type A individuals should follow a vegetarian diet.

> Blood Type B can enjoy meat, fruits and vegetables.

> Blood Type AB can eat pretty much anything that is applicable to those that belong in blood groups A and B.

> Blood Type O should stick to a diet that is high in protein, such as fish and meat.

Keep in mind that there is no fixed diet plan that can be followed by the general majority. People do not have the same basic nutritional needs. The differences among individuals, from their personalities to their unique blood chemistries, will dictate how their diet and exercise or fitness regimen should go.

Chapter 2 - Pros and Cons the Blood Type Diet

The Blood Type Diet, which advocates mirroring how our ancestors ate and in accordance with their blood types, is currently making waves, and it is even being followed by celebrities, most notable of which are Elizabeth Hurley, Sir Cliff Richard, Courtney Cox-Arquette and Cheryl Cole. But what are the benefits that can be derived from observing this diet? And what are its disadvantages?

Benefits of the Blood Type Diet

Weight Loss

Many are now turning to the Blood Type Diet in order for them to lose weight. Two of the reasons for weight gain are overeating and eating the wrong types of food. Using this diet to determine which foods are most suitable for you and which aren't will enable you to come up with a list of the foods to eat and the foods to avoid, thereby preventing you from overeating.

Instead of counting calories or keeping track of your carb intake, you will simply keep tabs on the foods that you eat. This is actually less complicated, and will allow you to still enjoy the foods that you love, provided they belong to the food group that your blood type should have.

Immune System Enhancement

Since this diet will specifically tell you which foods are most appropriate for your blood type, you can be sure that every food intake will contribute towards improving your immune system, increasing your immunity against certain diseases. It has been said that blood types play a defensive role against diseases, and eating the right types of food will definitely serve to strengthen your body's levels of defense.

Almost all the foods that we eat contain "lectin", which is a type of protein that can bind sugar molecules and with red blood cells. Too much lectin will then lead to the clumping of blood, and eventually to many types of illnesses. Since the blood type diet advocates eating only the foods that are compatible with your blood type, you will be preventing these lectins from wreaking havoc to your red blood cells and causing harm to your overall health.

Prevention and Cure of Certain Medical Conditions

Since the Blood Type Diet pretty much cuts out all processed and junk foods, you can be sure that you will be eating foods that are safe and will not induce adverse reactions as well as health conditions. They will be able to eliminate saturated fats from their diet and steer clear of the chemicals and substances added to highly processed foods.

Those who have tried following the Blood Type Diet observed that their allergies have decreased significantly. There are even people who claim that this diet helped lessen their asthma attacks as well as heartburn. People who often suffer from headaches and migraines also said their attacks have become less frequent since they decided to follow the Blood Type Diet.

Aside from the stated medical conditions, the other health risks that can be reduced by this diet include inflammatory disorders, blood clotting problems, diabetes and certain types of cancers.

Stress Management

Dealing with stress is also another benefit that can be obtained from this diet. When you are healthy because you ate the right types of food or, in this case, the foods that are compatible with your blood type, you will feel more able to handle even complex problems and even defuse difficult situations.

Energy Level Regulation

The Blood Type Diet also works in increasing one's energy levels, and regulating them. Some diets can effectively help increase your level of energy but they are unable to sustain it or keep it up. The result? The sudden drop will likely cause health problems as well as depression.

A General Sense of Well-Being

It's common sense, really. If you are in good shape, you are protected against illnesses and diseases, and you are able to handle stress while keeping your energy levels up, you will have a better sense of self and a brighter disposition to deal with everyday life.

Cons of the Blood Type Diet

Choice Restrictions

If you are serious about following the Blood Type Diet, you have to accept the fact that you may have to make sacrifices. There will hardly be any room for your personal tastes. It is unfortunate that blood type does not also dictate one's personal preferences, especially when it comes to food, then following the Blood Type Diet will not be difficult at all.

Let us say, for example, that you love eating carbs, and you always have a craving for meat. That is going to be a problem if you have the blood type A, since that blood group adheres to a vegetarian diet.

High Costs

Organic vegetables and foods do not come cheap, and some specialty food items that are recommended for certain blood types are also quite expensive. This diet also recommends the use of vitamins and other food supplements, and we are all aware that these also come with hefty price tags.

Conflicts with Certain Conditions

There is a need to first look into how the proposed diet will have an effect on a chronic condition that you currently have, if any. For instance, a Type O individual may already be suffering from diabetes and he is recommended to increase his protein intake. However, he is forbidden to consume chicken or dairy. This is quite a contradiction, which is why you have to first look into what your medical practitioner tells you before you launch on a diet in accordance with your blood type.

Deprivation of Key Nutrients

Since some major food groups are going to be cut out, you will be missing out on certain nutrients. Cutting out dairy products will mean you will not get the amount of calcium you need. You will then end up resorting to taking food supplements to make up for that lack, and the cost factor will figure greatly in the equation. Similarly, some may also suffer from lack of fiber because they had to cut out grains, beans or lentils from their diet.

Tedious Preparation

Getting on this diet means you will have your choices pared down considerably. That means you will have to prepare the food or dishes yourself, in order to adhere to the Blood Type Diet. Processed food and simple carbs are not at all recommended, too. This is going to be a problem for busy individuals who are always on the go and would prefer to have quick meals since they do not have enough time to prepare every meal.

Chapter 3 - Food Classifications as to Blood Type

As mentioned earlier, there are four blood groups, and the Blood Type Diet states that you should only eat the foods that are suited for your specific blood type. For purposes of the application of this diet, it is important to note that the pioneers of the Blood Type Diet named categorized all foods into 16 food groups.

1. Dairy (eggs, milk, cheese)

2. Meats (pork, poultry) and seafood (fish, shellfish)

3. Vegetables

4. Fruits

5. Legumes (beans, peas)

6. Oils and fats (i.e. linseed oil, olive oil, sesame oil, peanut oil)

7. Nuts and seeds

8. Baked goods (breads, muffins, crackers)

9. Cereals (barley, oats, corn flakes, puffed rice)

10. Grains (wheat, rye, millet)

11. Pasta (flour, buckwheat, noodles)

12. Juices (fruit juices and concentrates)

13. Condiments (dips, jams, jellies, pickles, relishes and dressings)

14. Spices (sauces, syrups, dried spices)

15. Herbal teas

16. Other beverages (coffee, other non-herbal teas, sodas, wine, beer, liquor)

What are the food classifications according to these four blood types?

Blood Type A, the "Cultivators"

People who are under this blood group are also known as the "cultivators", the "agrarian", or those that worked the earth, tilled the soil, planted crops and harvested them afterwards for consumption. The foods for this specific blood type include those that are obtained from plants and other plant sources. It is also frequently referred to as the "meat-free" diet.

Key points:

> Eat only fruits, vegetables, legumes and grains. Go for the organic and fresh ones since Type A individuals often have sensitive immune systems.

> Avoid meat (particularly red meat), and pile on protein-rich vegetables to make up for it.

> Avoid dairy products and wheat.

> ➤ Yoga, *tai chi* and other exercises that are low impact and involve only stretches and similar minor physical activities are recommended.

Blood Type B, the "Nomads"

These are the nomadic types of people, who have managed to develop high tolerance for different types of food while moving from place to place.

Key points:

> ➤ Eat a good mix of meat, fruits and vegetables.
>
> ➤ Dairy products are also acceptable.
>
> ➤ Avoid peanuts, corn, lentils, and even chicken.
>
> ➤ Walking, cycling and running are recommended exercises.

Blood Type AB, the "Enigma"

This is a rare blood group, and the few that belong to it can pretty much enjoy all the foods that people in blood groups A and B can eat. Meat and food from plant sources are definitely not a problem.

Key points:

> ➤ They can eat a wide variety of food, from meat, fish and other seafood, fruits, vegetables, and dairy.

> ➤ Avoid red meat, buckwheat, and some seeds.

> ➤ The recommended exercises can be a mix of yoga and running, since type AB individuals can handle both rigorous workouts and calming exercises.

Blood Type O, the "Hunters"

Majority of the population has blood type O, making it the most common blood group. Hunters are known to be constantly on the lookout for animals and wild beasts, which explains this blood group's affinity with meat.

Key points:

> ➤ The diet is mainly composed of meat, since it is a high-protein diet. However, keep carbs at a minimum.

> ➤ High amount of protein is required for people with blood type O to lose weight.

> ➤ Avoid grains, as they may cause more harm than good to the health.

> ➤ Aerobic exercises are recommended.

Is the Blood Type Diet Restrictive?

This is one question that will understandably be asked by many. Does this mean that you should only limit the foods you eat to the ones that are allowed for your blood type?

The answer is NO.

If your goal is to lose weight or to improve your overall health, it is not advisable to completely cut out specific foods. Striking the right balance is still key to any weight loss plan. Eat any type of food; it's just a matter of taking them in moderation and managing the portions accordingly.

Chapter 4 - Blood Type Diet for Weight Loss and Overall Health

The main benefits of the Blood Type Diet (and the main reasons it is favored by many) are weight loss and improved overall health. True, it has a lot more to offer, but these two are the main reasons why this diet is favored by many.

Weight Loss

This diet recognizes the variability in metabolism of people with different blood types, and recommends the foods that will ensure they are absorbed by the body without piling on the fats or the unwanted weight.

Any weight loss plan will surely benefit from having the Blood Type Diet incorporated into it. By eating only the foods that are compatible with your blood type, you will have better chances of losing weight, and keeping it off.

When you decide to integrate this diet into your weight loss plan, there are several things that you must first know and fully accept.

- People have varying rates of metabolism. Some simply metabolize faster than others, and this is also dependent on the macronutrients being processed in one's system.

- People have varying responses to certain types of food. There are people that develop adverse reactions to some foods, such as dairy. Meanwhile, there are also those that have no issues whatsoever with whatever they eat. For example, some are lactose-intolerant, while others are hypoglycemic, which means they have to watch their blood sugar levels at all times and eat only those that will not cause any sudden or irregular spikes or drops.

- People may already have preexisting medical conditions, allergies or food intolerances that prohibit them from enjoying certain types of food, even if their blood type is compatible with them.

- A huge reason why you weigh more than you should is because you eat too much. Sticking to a specific diet, such as the Blood Type Diet, will help you choose only the foods that will be most beneficial to you and will be compatible with your body's specific digestive needs.

Good Overall Health

The Blood Type Diet works to improve your overall health by targeting your first defense against sickness and other diseases: your immune system. And that is where the blood and blood type comes in. It is the main driving force that can control the various factors that can compromise the immune system, such as bacteria, viruses, and other harmful chemicals.

The Immune System's Role

The immune system is considered to be the main barrier between your body and that of outside invaders that can compromise your health. That is its main role: to protect you from these harmful agents.

How does it do it, you ask?

The immune system operates just like a sensor, sniffing out and identifying *antigens*, or those substances that act as chemical markers. It is these antigens that the immune system reacts to, and it does that by producing antibodies that are specifically meant to battle that identified antigen.

Antigens is actually any substance that triggers a reaction from the immune system, so they may also be foreign substances found in the environment, such as chemicals, viruses or bacteria. But antigens may also be formed inside the body, usually in the form of tissue cells and bacterial toxins. As such, you can expect the human body to already have antigens, and each blood type, with its own unique chemical structure, also has its own unique antigens.

Upon detection of these antigens, the immune system then produces antibodies, which will specifically target those substances that they have been designed to destroy. The antibody will then stick to the antigen, and *agglutination* takes place. This means that the substances or antigens are clumped together, and the body will then find it easier to eject or eliminate them.

But the agglutination process is not without complications. When blood agglutinates or sticks together, you will likely feel fatigue and experience headaches, digestive problems and different skin issues, to name just a few.

No thanks to the presence of *lectins*, or proteins found in certain types of foods, the agglutination process may take place faster, or it may even take place even when it shouldn't. Of the lectins ingested by the body, 95% are eliminated due to the action of the immune system. The remaining 5%, however, remains in the body, making its way to the different organs, tissues and cells through the bloodstream. That is where they inflict damage. By eating according to your bloody type, you are bolstering your immune system to get rid of as much lectin as it could - possibly even 100%! - so you will be healthier.

This is where the variability in blood types comes in. It is possible that a person will eat lectin-rich food that is incompatible with his blood type. As a result, agglutination may take place in the part of the body specifically targeted by the lectin. This means that healthy cells are marked as foreign substances, clumped together, and eliminated from the body. This would then lead to certain types of illnesses and complications.

Specific Health Benefits of the Blood Type Diet

You were given a quick run through of the health benefits of the Blood Type Diet earlier. This time, we will try to go into more detail and list down how you can achieve overall good health with this diet.

- It effectively prevents obesity.

- It allows you to get rid of body fats and toxins that are often the cause of various illnesses and diseases.

- It bolsters your immunity to protect you against common infections, viruses and bacteria.

- It effectively kills the free radicals that cause the rapid deterioration of cells and aging.

- It promotes healthier skin, hair and bones. Acne breakouts and other skin problems are addressed directly by eating the right foods for you, depending on your blood type.

- It reduces the risks of the following conditions:

  - Various types of cancer

  - Various cardiovascular diseases

  - Liver problems

  - Diabetes

Chapter 5 - Blood Type Diet for Blood Group A

In Chapter 3, you were given an overview of the food classifications and recommended exercises for each of the four blood groups. It is time to delve deeper into each blood type.

The "cultivators", or those that belong to the blood group A, are first on the list. They are often described as the hardworking lot. Their competitive nature often turns them into perfectionists, and they seek excellence in almost everything they do.

Type A women are known to have higher fertility rates, which explains the need for them to eat food that will address fertility. As for susceptibility to certain diseases, people with blood type A are more prone to microbial infections.

Among the four blood groups, Type A are said to be more susceptible to stress, and that is due to the high levels of *cortisol*, the stress hormone, in their body.

Type A individuals can derive the following benefits from the Blood Type Diet:

- Weight loss

- Reduced risk of anemia and disorders involving the gall bladder and the liver

- Reduced risk of heart diseases and Type 1 Diabetes

Foods to Eat

Generally, Type A individuals will derive more benefits if they follow a diet composed of fruits, grains and vegetables. In fact, in most cases, this blood group is recommended to observe a vegetarian diet, and stick only to natural and fresh foods.

> - Use vegetable oils instead of animal fats, corn oil or sesame oil.

> - The best fruits for this diet include apples, avocados, berries, figs, peaches, pears, and plums.

> - Choose vegetables such as artichokes, broccoli, carrots and other greens.

> - Soy products are also good additions to your diet for their soy protein content.

> - Supplements are highly encouraged in order to make up for the loss of some food products that have them. Examples include Calcium (from milk and other dairy products), Iron, and Vitamins A and E.

Foods to Avoid

Meats and dairy foods are the major causes of weight gain among Type A individuals. As much as possible, reduce the intake or consumption of the following, as they will not do you any favors, and may even harm your health:

> - Milk, cheese, and other dairy products

- ➢ Meat products (specifically red meat) since they, in general, are more difficult to digest for Type As. Type A individuals have high digestive enzymes for carbohydrates, but not for animal proteins.

- ➢ Teas and beverages such as black tea, cayenne tea, corn silk tea, red clover tea, beer, liquor, and soda, since alcohol and caffeine will only increase cortisol levels, which are already high among Type As to begin with

- ➢ Legumes, nuts, beans and seeds, such as cashews, pistachios, and walnuts

- ➢ Wheat and other wheat-based products, such as whole wheat bread, wheat-bran muffins, and multi-grain bread

- ➢ Dips and sauces such as ketchup, mayonnaise and Worcestershire sauce

- ➢ Liquor and other alcoholic beverages

- ➢ Keep caffeine and sugar at a minimum

Another great advice to Type A individuals is to avoid fast foods and processed foods altogether. Since they also have sensitive immune systems, it is important to keep it nourished at all times. Skipping meals is a no-no, and make every effort to avoid stressful situations, including environments with too much noise, or even extreme weather conditions.

Recommended Exercises

Type A individuals are, as mentioned before, prone to stress. Therefore, they will benefit best from the following calming exercises:

> ➢ Yoga or other forms of meditation

> ➢ Tai chi

> ➢ Pilates

> ➢ Isometric exercises

Steer clear of high intensity exercises, since they will only increase your cortisol levels. Type As that perform intense exercises tend to suffer from muscle fatigue and stiffness afterwards.

Chapter 6 - Blood Type Diet for Blood Group B

Those that belong under this category are known for their patience and their laidback nature. They are also able to adapt more easily to various circumstances and environments. The key words to their specific diet are "less meat, more dairy".

This blood group is said to possess robust immune systems as well as a tolerant digestive system. They also tend to have higher immunity against allergies, although give them the wrong food and the allergic reactions will be more apparent. Those who belong to this blood group also have a high tendency to be afflicted with pancreatic cancer, which requires more attention to building up their immune systems.

Observing the Blood Type Diet will help Type B individuals derive the following advantages:

- Weight loss

- Reduced risk of autoimmune disorders such as lupus, multiple sclerosis (MS) and Lou Gehrig's disease

- Reduced risk of chronic fatigue syndrome

- Reduced risk of Type 1 Diabetes

Foods to Eat

It is safe to say that this blood group has the least number of dietary restrictions. They have more variety to choose from; it's just a matter of keeping everything balanced.

Type B individuals will need to focus more on boosting and strengthening their immune systems, if they want to lose weight or remain healthy. They should also focus on regulating their insulin and blood sugar levels to keep them from fluctuating wildly. In order to do that, the following foods are encouraged.

> ➢ Include more fruits and fresh greens to your diet, and try to consume them up to five times a day. Leafy greens, bananas, grapes, pineapple and plums will do very nicely.

> ➢ Dairy is all right. Thus, eggs, milk, milk-based beverages and other low-fat dairy products should be consumed.

> ➢ Lean meats, but only in limited amounts, and only specific types of meat, such as turkey and lamb.

> ➢ Add olive oil and flaxseed oil to your foods.

> ➢ Oatmeal, rice bran and millet are good breakfast fare.

> ➢ Several types of seafoods that are high in protein.

> ➢ Stick to water, green tea and natural fruit juices. You may drink beer, wine, or caffeine, but only in small amounts.

Foods to Avoid

Steer clear of the following:

- ➢ Gluten- and carbohydrate-rich foods, such as wheat, corn, wheat, lentils, and peanuts, since they slow down metabolism and promote the storage of fat in the body

- ➢ Chicken and other poultry products

- ➢ Peanut, corn and other corn-based products

- ➢ Shellfish, crab, lobster and shrimps.

Recommended Exercises

If your blood type is B, you are better off performing rigorous exercises such as hiking, walking, cycling and jogging. Several rounds of golf or sets of tennis won't hurt, either. Notice how these physical exercises place great emphasis on having mental balance. However, compared to the exercises for blood type O individuals, keep your pace at a moderate level.

- ➢ Moderate walking, hiking and jogging

- ➢ Tennis games

- ➢ Cycling

- ➢ Golf

- ➢ Low impact cardio exercises

- ➢ Resistance training

True to their nomadic nature, Type Bs prefer to do things in packs or in groups, so joining group classes or exercises will be a good idea.

32

Chapter 7 - Blood Type Diet for Blood Group AB

The enigmatic group under Blood Type AB is pretty much a combination of types A and B, so they are considered to be the chosen few. Not only are they allowed to enjoy a larger variety of foods, but they are also known to have very strong immune systems. That does not mean, however, that they are completely impervious to diseases or other medical conditions. They still need to eat right in order to stay healthy.

Of course, it is also natural that the bad points of both A and B blood groups are also shared by the AB group. The most common health conditions that people under this blood group suffer include anemia, heart disease and certain types of cancer, such as pancreatic cancer. They also tend to have sensitive digestive systems, despite the fact that they have more food options. With the right food and exercise, their immune system will be at its strongest to ward off these conditions.

With the help of the Blood Type Diet, Type AB individuals can get the following benefits:

- Weight loss

- Reduced risks of anemia and heart diseases

- Reduced risks of developing cancer

Foods to Eat

As mentioned earlier, Type AB individuals can eat the foods that Types A and B are allowed to consume. They may also choose to eat frequent meals, but in small portions or servings.

> ➢ Fruits, vegetables and grains are greatly encouraged. In fact, it would be best if vegetables are consumed daily. The recommended fruits include apricots, cherries, grapefruit, grapes, kiwi, lemons, pineapples, and plums.

> ➢ Seafood and other iodine-rich foods are encouraged.

> ➢ Certain types of meat (lamb, turkey, or mutton) are also recommended.

> ➢ Include tofu and other soy foods.

> ➢ They can also handle eggs, milk and other dairy products.

> ➢ Drink coffee and green tea. Red wine is recommended, but keep it to one glass per day.

Foods to Avoid

If you are Type AB, you should limit your meat consumption and go for substitutes instead. Tofu is one excellent (and healthier) alternative to meats. The foods that should be avoided at all costs include:

> ➢ Red meat, cured meat and smoked meat

> Poultry products, since chicken has high lectin content

> Red beans and kidney beans

> Corn

> Peppers, oranges and other acidic foods that will counter the alkaline in your stomach

> Ketchup and vinegar

> Caffeine and alcohol

Recommended Exercises

Type AB individuals will feel comfortable performing any of the exercises suited for both types A and B. That means they should look into including yoga, pilates, golf, running and walking in their exercise regimen. Swimming and dancing are also highly recommended.

However, try to avoid high intensity exercises, since Type Abs are prone to experience stiffness in the muscles and joints after a high-power session.

Chapter 8 - Blood Type Diet for Blood Group O

A great majority of the world's population fall under the blood group O. Known for their great leadership skills and organization, these individuals are said to have the strongest immune systems among the four groups. They also have a lower risk for heart disease. However, the risk for developing stomach ulcers is significantly higher, and you will find that most sufferers of arthritis and gout are Type Os. That means grains, potatoes and other foods that can cause joint inflammations are prohibited.

When it comes to stress responses, this blood group cultivates the "fight or flight" response, which explains how their body produces adrenaline in great amounts. It is the Type A individuals who easily succumb to stress; Type O individuals do not easily fall at the first signs of stress, but when they do, the recovery period is longer. This is because the overproduction of adrenaline means it will take a longer time for their adrenaline levels to go down to acceptable levels.

The Blood Type Diet will provide the following benefits to Type O individuals:

- Weight loss

- Prevention of blood clotting disorder

- Prevention of inflammatory diseases, such as arthritis, asthma, hypothyroidism, and asthma

Foods to Eat

If you notice, the Type A diet closely resembles the vegetarian diet. In the case of the Type O diet, it is akin to the Paleo diet. Some even say that it is a slight variation of the Atkins Diet.

Type O individuals should pay more attention to keeping their immune system in top condition, and they can do that by eating right. The equation would be "high-protein, and low-dairy". The high stomach acid content found in Type O individuals allows them to consume and easily metabolize meat and animal protein. Thus, they may eat the foods listed below.

- Meat, fish, fruits and vegetables are essential components of the Type O's diet

- Iodine-rich seafood, such as bluefish, cod, halibut, mackerel, pike, salmon, sea kelp, snapper, sole, sturgeon, and swordfish, and trout, since they increase hormone production and regulates thyroid functions.

- Lean meats, such as beef, lamb, mutton, veal and venison

- Green leafy vegetables, such as broccoli, kale and spinach, should be prioritized

- Fruits high in alkaline content, such as different types of berries and plums.

Foods to Avoid

While ensuring that protein levels are high, these foods must be avoided.

- ➢ All dairy products and gluten-rich foods. Wheat and gluten are considered to be the main culprits when it comes to weight gain among Type O individuals.

- ➢ Carbohydrate-rich foods such as cereals, breads and legumes

- ➢ Peanut, corn and other corn-based products, wheat and other wheat-based products

- ➢ Beans and legumes, such as lentils and kidney beans

- ➢ Cabbage, cauliflower and other vegetables belonging to the Brassica family, since they inhibit thyroid function

Recommended Exercises

For blood type O individuals, who are on the 'strong and athletic' side, the more intense, demanding, and vigorous the exercises, the better. That is because they are more prone to weight gain (which is partly the reason why carbohydrates are discouraged).

High intensity exercises will also help in speeding up the recovery process due to the overproduction of adrenaline. They are excellent mood boosters, so you'll be able to bring down your stress levels faster.

Therefore, incorporate the following high intensity workouts in your fitness program:

- ➢ Running or jogging uphill, on long distances, or on a treadmill

- ➢ Weight training

- Interval training, or High Intensity Interval Training (HIIT)

- Biking or cycling

- Swimming

- Plyometrics

- Martial arts

- Aerobics

- Contact sports

Make sure you work out regularly in order to stay fit. This will also ensure that stomach problems and ulcers - which are common for Type O individuals – will also be regulated.

Thanks

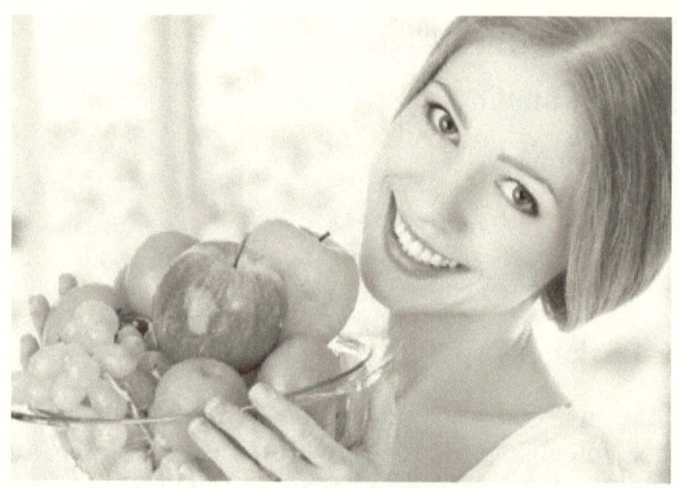

Thank you again for downloading this book "Eat Right For Your Blood Type*: A Guide to Healthy Blood Type Diet, Understand What to Eat According to Your Blood Type*"!

I hope this book was able to help you to learn more about the Eating Right for Your Blood Type Guide and the Blood Type Diet what it is, how it works, and what it can do for you.

The next step is to go about finding out what your blood type is and formulating a nutritional diet and exercise regime that suits your specific blood type. Whatever your goal is - to lose weight, to look good, or to be healthier - you can definitely try the Blood Type Diet for yourself and start reaping the results in no time at all!

Finally, if you enjoyed this book, then I'd like to ask you for a favor, would you be kind enough to leave a review for this book on Amazon? It'd be greatly appreciated!

Please leave a review for this book on Amazon!

41

Thank you and good luck!

WaraWaran R.